"Beloved, I wish above all things that thou mayest prosper and be in health, even as thy soul prospereth."
3 John 1:2 (KJV)

100 Health Secrets

Dr. Byron G. Jackson

ISBN: 1516803698
ISBN 13: 9781516803699

Most of Dr. Byron G. Jackson's products are available at special quantity discounts for bulk purchase for sale promotions, premiums, fundraising, and educational needs.
For details, contact:

Think Large International
P.O. Box 201852
Shaker Heights, OH 44120
770-714-1157: Phone
888-558-0456: Fax
bgjackson@hotmail.com: email
www.DrByrongJackson.com: website

100 HEALTH SECRETS™

This book was printed in the United States of America.

ISBN: 1516803698
ISBN 13: 9781516803699

**Other national books by
Dr. Byron G. Jackson:**

*STAND TALL, DREAM BIG, THINK LARGE,
I DARE YOU!*
We Can All Be Champions

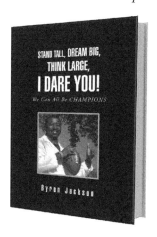

THE WAY I DID IT
Lose Weight & Look Great Naturally

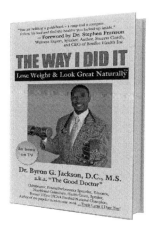

Note to the Reader (disclaimer)

Please be advised that this book is solely for informational and educational purposes only. It is also important to note that this book should not in any way be regarded as a substitute for professional health care or medical treatment. The statements in this book have not been evaluated by the Food and Drug Administration, and therefore the information contained in it should not be used or construed to be used to diagnose, treat, cure, or prevent any disease or illness. Do not delay seeking professional health-care advice based on information in this book.

The statements in this book contain opinions and ideas that the author has endeavored to make as accurate and reliable as possible at the time of writing/publication. However, research is sometimes subject to interpretation and evolves; therefore, the information, suggestions, recommendations, and/or conclusions presented herein may differ from those found in other sources. It should also be acknowledged that the nature of your body and/or health condition is complex and unique, so you should always consult your health-care professional and licensed doctor before beginning any exercise, nutrition, or supplementation program. By maintaining possession of this book, you agree in good faith that you are solely responsible for your own health and that neither the author nor the publisher nor any third party mentioned shall be liable, nor do they accept responsibly for any claims of adverse effects, whether directly or indirectly, based on information, sources suggestions, recommendations, and/or conclusions contained herein.

Remember to always consult with your health-care provider and/or doctor before using or starting any new health-care regimen.

Contents

One

Broccoli is a vegetable I consider important. Not only does it fight cancer, but it also outranks oranges in vitamin C and can have just as much calcium as milk. To receive the most benefits broccoli has to offer, avoid eating "broccoli mush." Broccoli mush is when the broccoli has been cooked so long that it becomes wilted and mushy (hence the name broccoli mush). Instead, try eating broccoli cooked as little as possible. One way to do this is to break up the broccoli and place it on a salad or in a smoothie. And on the days you prefer having broccoli as a side dish, lightly steam it on the stove (not the microwave). When you do cook it, be sure it remains slightly firm and crisp. Cooking broccoli–and any other vegetable, for that matter—until it is soft and mushy kills most of its nutrients.

Two

SEVEN SUPERFOODS AND THEIR BENEFITS

- watermelon:
  relaxes blood vessels
  improves heart function
  improves immune function

- blueberries ⎤
  blackberries ⎥
  cranberries ⎦
  slow some cancer growth
  improve brain function
  improve muscle tone
  improve balance

- olive oil
  helps with inflammation

- tomatoes
  improve skin texture
  may reduce cancer and heart disease risks

- fish
  helps lower risk of Alzheimer's and strokes

- almonds ⌝
  walnuts ⌟

  improve heart function
  improve brain function
  help with inflammation

- red grapes

  help with inflammation
  help with blood clots

Three

To obtain and maintain a healthy diet, eat a piece of fruit, salad, or soup before your meal. In a study measuring how much people ate, it was observed that people who ate an apple fifteen minutes before their lunch ate 190 fewer calories.

Four

As much as it has been said, breakfast really is the most important meal of the day. Skipping breakfast has been linked to mood swings, weight gain, and a variety of other health conditions. Just remember, you cannot drive a car without fuel, and your body cannot and will not properly function without its fuel—food. You only have one true place to live, and that it is your body, so you have to take care of it. Before you leave your home in the morning, make it a priority to properly fuel your body by eating breakfast.

Five

It has been theorized that not eating breakfast regularly may increase your cholesterol level and your chances of heart disease and diabetes.

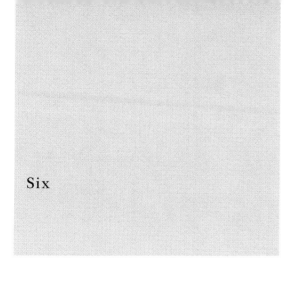

Six

Eating fried foods more than once per week may increase the risk of prostate cancer by 33 percent.

Seven

Avoiding these foods may help you experience a better level of health and increase your performance:

- wheat
- processed sugar
- white flour
- processed salt
- artificial sweeteners

Eight

After cooking rice, refrigerate it within two hours and throw it away after the third day.

Nine

A void buying ice cream with freezer frost because it may have been defrosted and then refrozen, causing it to possibly reach the temperature danger zone (the range at which bacteria can grow).

Ten

Fish are not meant to be raised on a farm and should be caught in the wild. Wild fish are better to eat than farmed fish because they are less crowded in the water. When fish are confined to one area (in the case of some farmed fish), their chances of being more toxic is increased because they are eating and using the bathroom in the same vicinity.

Eleven

A food rule to remember is to never eat things that cause you discomfort. I once heard someone say that eating a certain food gave them a headache. Sometimes your body whispers to you, and sometimes it yells. If you continuously eat things that do not agree with your body, you will build up a tolerance for it and eventually desensitize the whispering. The problem with doing this is that you force your body to tolerate something that is bad for it. Eventually it will yell, and it may yell in the form of serious health issues. Listen to your body.

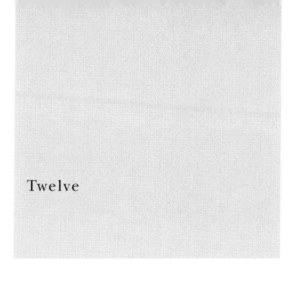

Twelve

If chocolate is your snack of choice, choose dark chocolate over milk chocolate and white chocolate (also referred to as "fake chocolate"). Dark chocolate contains antioxidants that help combat and defend against potentially harmful toxins, cells, and molecules such as free radicals. But all dark chocolates are not created equally. Look for those that have cocoa/cacao percentages of seventy or higher (which is usually printed in bold letters on the front wrapper) and those that do not have *high fructose corn syrup* or *partially hydrogenated oils* listed on their ingredients label.

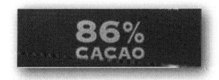

Thirteen

It is common restaurant practice to receive water with a lemon wedge at sit-down restaurants and ice in your cup at fast-food restaurants. Unfortunately, these common courtesies may be affecting your health. Studies have shown that lemon wedges at some "popular family restaurants" were contaminated from not being properly washed, and at some fast-food restaurants, the ice was more contaminated than toilet water from the machine not being regularly cleaned. As a suggestion, you may want to ask for no ice and no lemon wedge or lemon wedge on the side the next time you eat out. Otherwise, your health maybe affected.

Fourteen

Drinking three or four alcoholic beverages a day increases a man's risk of mouth, neck, and throat cancer and makes him twice as likely to have high blood pressure and develop liver cirrhosis.

Fifteen

All fats are not bad. Your brain requires fat to function. Your body uses fat for energy and to absorb vitamins and nutrients. Good fats are olive oil, coconut oil, avocados, nuts, egg yolks (from good, healthy chickens), and omega-3 fatty acids like fish oil. Some of the most common bad fats are saturated fats, trans fats, margarine, and shortening.

Sixteen

One of the key reasons processed foods (fast foods and premade/prepackaged foods) are bad is because of the amount of salt they contain. On average the recommended amount of salt per day is about a teaspoon or less. Our diets, however, consists of about three times that, which is mostly derived from processed foods. When extra salt is in your body, your heart has to pump harder, ultimately increasing your chances of stroke, heart disease, and high blood pressure.

Seventeen

Over a seventeen-year period, data was collected regarding the health and lifestyle choices of 43,727 people. The results determined that "coffee intake was positively associated with all-cause mortality in men." Drinking more than twenty-eight cups of coffee a week increased a person's risk of death by 21 percent, and in both men and women younger than fifty-five, the risk of death was greater than 50 percent.

Eighteen

At some point or another, you have probably overly excited your taste buds by feasting at an all-you-can-eat buffet. If so, you are aware of how easy it is to over-eat because of the vast array of foods available. During a restaurant study, it was observed that "normal weight" customers and overweight customers behaved differently at all-you-can-eat buffets. Try these behavioral strategies the next time you're at a buffet to avoid overeating:

- Eat at a booth instead of a table.
- Sit with your back or side facing the buffet while you eat.
- Survey the entire selection of food before preparing your plate.
- Use smaller plates if possible.
- Put your napkin on your lap instead of on the table or tucked into your shirt.
- Make a conscious effort to chew your food several times before swallowing.

Nineteen

To prevent botulism (food poising) in kids, never give them honey under the age of one.

Twenty

Never ignore hip pain and limping in children. If you notice a child complaining of hip pain or limping, don't dismiss it as growing pains; it could be a serious bone or circulation problem that could affect the rest of his or her life if not treated promptly. If a child complains of hip pain and limping, contact the doctor immediately.

Twenty-One

For the song "Greatest Love of All," songwriters Michael Masser and Linda Creed wrote: "I believe the children are our future. Teach them well and let them lead the way. Show them all the beauty they possess inside."

A starting point to bringing this timeless melody to fruition is to limit the amount of soft drinks children consume. Researchers noted that children who drank more than three sodas a day were twice as likely to be violent and aggressive.

Twenty-Two

Obesity has been known to affect men and women of all races and creeds, but unfortunately children are being affected as well. When fat accumulates in the body, the liver swells and develops scarring similar to what happens to the livers of those who drink heavily. When a child's body endures this kind of stress, it increases their chances of needing liver replacement surgery in their adult years. Childhood obesity may be combated by simply seeing to it that children receive adequate rest.

Researchers found that when third graders slept less than nine hours and forty-five minutes, their chances of being obese in sixth grade significanty increased. It was also noted that every extra hour third graders sleep per night reduces their chances of being obese in sixth grade by 40 percent.

Sleep or a lack thereof alters hormones that control appetite regulation, and less sleep equals tired children, and tired children are less apt to exercise and engage in high levels of physical activity.

Twenty-Three

When necessary, cesarean births (C-sections) can be the answer to the prayers of expecting parents. However, this process should not be used at the expense of convenience or cosmetic vanity. Unknown to some, C-sections can pose dangerous health problems like infections, blood loss, blood clotting in the legs, blood clotting in the lungs, headaches, vomiting, nausea, constipation, breathing problems, and possible injury to the newborn. This issue is so serious that hospitals that deliver more than eleven hundred babies a year have been urged to "actively work toward reducing C-sections."

Twenty-Four

Breastfeeding for at least six months can reduce a child's chances of recurrent infections and pneumonia. A *New York Times* article stated that if a child stops breastfeeding after four months, the chance of infection is higher than that of daycare attendance or being exposed to smoke.

Twenty-Five

When it comes to health, I prefer focusing on adding good things rather than getting rid of bad things. Unfortunately, for women who are pregnant or planning for pregnancy, that option may not be as much of a luxury. In a study conducted by Kaiser Permanente Division of Research, caffeine (whether from coffee, tea, or soft drinks) was shown to increase the risk of miscarriage by two times. This is not to say that caffeine is completely bad, but consuming two or more cups of coffee or five cans of soda per day while pregnant can be very bad for the mother and her unborn child.

Twenty-Six

To some, tattoos are what art is to others, but tattoos may carry with them higher prices. During childbirth it is a regular custom for women to receive a lower-back injection known as an epidural, which helps desensitize the pain. As it turns out, some doctors are concerned about administering epidurals to women with lower-back tattoos because of the chances of transferring ink from the tattoo to the spinal canal via the injection needle.

If you do have a tattoo, removing it may not be the best thing either. Tattoo removal can also pose serious threats because the heat that is used to remove tattoos can create a chemical reaction that results in cancer cells being absorbed in the body. Also, it is important to notify your doctor if you have tattoos because if you need to undergo medical testing like MRI scans, the metal(s) contained in some tattoo inks may cause areas of your body to swell and burn.

Twenty-Seven

An NYU Langone Medical Center study revealed that tattoos shaded with red or black ink have been linked to health complications that have lasted as long as several years.

Twenty-Eight

One of the scariest problems facing us on a day-to-day basis is thinking that our health is OK when it is not. It has been said that only about 10 percent of our nerves are designed to make us feel pain, so waiting for an ache or pain to appear before you see your doctor for a checkup is not a good idea. By the time you finally feel an ache or pain, it may be a late indication that a problem has been lurking that you just did not know about. For example, if you have ever had a cavity or toothache, I am sure your dentist informed you that the problem had been developing for a while before you ever felt the pain. You just did not know it. So make it a point to have regular consistent checkups with your doctor and never, ever ignore discomforting symptoms—because health issues don't just go away.

Twenty-Nine

When scheduling your annual physical (medical exam), be sure to schedule a "complete comprehensive exam," also referred to as an "executive physical." There are three other physicals: a problem-focused exam, an expanded problem-focused exam, and a detailed exam, but none of them are more thorough than a complete comprehensive exam (in which you are examined from top to bottom). The complete comprehensive exam covers everything from chest X-rays, heart tests, stress tests, blood work, and so on. Keep in mind that the complete comprehensive exam requires more of the doctor's time, and the doctor's staff will have to schedule your appointment accordingly. Be sure to use the words *executive physical* or *complete comprehensive exam* when you schedule your next examination appointment.

Thirty

When receiving care from new hospital residents, be certain that there is an attending supervisor present, especially during the months of July and August (*the July phenomenon*). Some say that during the months of July and August, when new residents join the staff, a percentage of medical quality and productivity decrease.

Thirty-One

Always get a second opinion when it comes to a significant health diagnosis or treatment. Sometimes a test can render a positive result but actually be false, known as a false-positive. It has been estimated that 20 to 30 percent of heart tests have resulted in false-positives. Our health-care system is good, but just like anything else, it's not always 100 percent accurate.

Always remember that you have the final say when it comes to your health, and requesting a second opinion is in no way an offense to your doctor because your doctor works for you. Nowadays, some health-care facilities have made it so convenient that you can even request a second opinion over the Internet.

Thirty-Two

In some instances, surgery is necessary and very much necessary, but in some conditions like hernias, surgery may not be an immediate requirement. It has been suggested that if a man's symptoms are considered mild or nonexistent, a better option might be nonsurgical treatment. In nonemergency situations, always consult with your doctor as to alternatives that may be suitable to your specific condition.

Thirty-Three

When in doubt, never put heat on a joint; use ice. Without the supervision of a qualified health professional, heating pads and compresses may feel good but may cause more harm than benefit. Heat is usually used to relax muscles, but when placed on a joint outside of the proper time frame, swelling and inflammation can develop and prolong the healing and recovery process. While ice is usually a safer bet, icing too long can also be detrimental. It has been suggested that icing an injured area for ten minutes three times a day is sufficient as long as at least one hour has elapsed between icing. Ice is usually always the therapy of choice in the initial injury phase because it helps reduce inflammation and helps speeds up the recovery process.

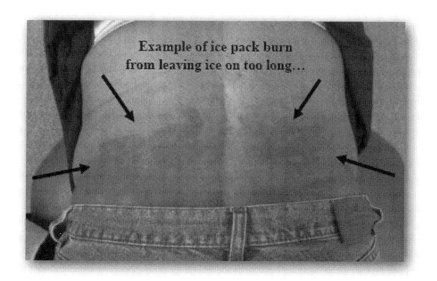

NOTE

Prepackaged ice packs tend to be colder than ice because of the chemicals inside them, and that is why it may take longer for prepackaged ice packs to defrost. Ice in a sandwich bag begins to defrost and melt the moment it's taken out of the freezer. When icing you should always wrap ice packs in a paper towel prior to placing them on your skin.

Injury Time Frame	Clinical Description	Modalities	Rationale
Injury to Day 2	• Swelling • Painful to touch • Pain upon motion	Ice	Decreases swelling and pain
Day 3	• Painful to touch • Pain upon motion	Ice and Heat	Ice for swelling and pain; and heat to mildly increase circulation
Day 4 to Day 6	• Swelling Decreases • Injured area warm • Discoloration • Painful to touch • Pain upon motion	Ice	Decreases swelling and pain
Day 7	• Swelling • Slight pain upon motion	Functional Exercises	Restores range of motion and strength

Thirty-Four

In an effort to promote quality and safety before and after surgery, the Joint Commission's "Speak Up: Help Avoid Mistakes in Your Surgery" campaign recommends:

- asking your doctor if there are any medications (including over-the-counter drugs) you should avoid before your surgery;
- asking your doctor if it is safe to eat or drink before your surgery;
- asking your doctor if you should trim your nails and remove nail polish before your surgery;
- asking someone you trust to escort you to and from the facility where you are having your surgery;
- asking someone you trust to be with you at the surgical facility;
- showering and washing your hair before arriving for surgery;
- not wearing makeup;
- not bringing jewelry, money, or other valuables with you to the surgical facility;

- reading the surgical facility's *Informed Consent Form* carefully to make sure you understand the kind of surgery you will have and the surgical risks before you sign it;
- informing your doctor or nurse about your pain after surgery;
- asking questions about the medication(s) you are given after surgery and their side effects;
- informing your caregiver about any allergies you have to medicines after surgery;
- talking to your doctor or nurse after surgery about any questions you might have regarding your medication before taking it;
- asking how long the liquid in your IV should take to run out and telling the nurse if it seems to be dripping too fast or too slow;
- asking your doctor if you will need therapy or medicines after you leave the surgical facility; and
- asking when you can resume daily activities like work, exercise, and travel.

Thirty-Five

DOCTORS AND THEIR
AREAS OF SPECIALTY

Type of Doctor	General Specialty
cardiologist	heart
chiropractor	spine and nervous system, correction of pinched nerves
endocrinologist	gland diseases including diabetes mellitus
internist	internal diseases like high blood pressure and hepatitis
gastroenterologist	digestion: ulcers, diverticulitis, Crohn's disease, ulcerative colitis, etc.
neurologist	neurological disorders: MS, Parkinson's, ALS, Brown–Sequard, cauda equina, etc.

orthopedist	musculoskeletal: tears and fractures
physiatrist	rehabilitation
psychologist	life issues and mental health
physical therapist	mobility, muscular function
podiatrist	foot, ankle, and lower extremity

According to a national poll, the highest-ranking fear regarding getting old was not being alone, health-insurance cost, dying, being dependent, or income problems. The biggest fear was health problems. You only have one true place to live, and that is your body; so you must take care of it.

Thirty-Six

When you have your blood pressure taken, you should be sitting in a chair and not lying down. Having your blood pressure taken while you sit in a chair and having at least five minutes' rest beforehand can affect your blood pressure reading by as much as fourteen points. This simple change can possibly be the difference between being diagnosed with high blood pressure and not.

Also see to it that when your blood pressure is taken, it is done on both arms.

Thirty-Seven

Some diseases are deadly because of their silent symptoms. Cardiovascular disease for example kills about five hundred thousand women a year in America. That means that women have a higher risk of dying from heart disease, hypertension, or stroke more than all other cancers combined. A diet high in vegetables, fruit, lean meat, and healthy fats, along with regular exercise and relaxation, can help reduce that likelihood and help you live a healthier, happier, longer, more productive life.

Thirty-Eight

If you notice any of the following after having your blood taken, go to the nearest hospital because you may be experiencing nerve damage or internal invisible bleeding from an injection injury:

- an electric shock in your arm or hand
- prolonged bleeding
- extended arm or hand pain

Thirty-Nine

HealthcareBlueBook.com is a free website that provides health-care pricing averages in your area.

Forty

The cost of health-care can be devastating. According to one statistic, 62 percent of bankruptcies filed in America were health related. If you are over your head in medical bills, know that sometimes hospitals will provide discounts of up to 40 percent to uninsured patients. Simply contact the hospital's financial-assistance office, uncompensated services department, or office of patient accounts and inquire about financial-assistance options. Be very frank, and explain that you are unable to pay the balance of your medical bills. If you are favored enough to receive a reduction in your bill, politely ask the representative to mail you a copy of the reduction.

Forty-One

Prior to taking medication, it has been recommended that you inquire as to whether your medication is FDA approved for your specific complaint. Previously, one out of seven common drugs were prescribed/taken for uses outside of what they were approved for. This may have happened because of the assumption that because a drug is FDA approved then it is OK to be taken. However, approved drugs are approved for specific uses and should be taken for those uses only.

- Of these following drugs, almost two-thirds of them were misprescribed for uses the FDA did not approve them for:

Prescription Name:	Brand Name:	Approved For:
Gabepentin	Neurontin	Seizures and Epilepsy
Risperidone	Risperdal	Schizophrenia, Mania, and Bipolar Disorder
Temazepan	Restoril	Short-Term Insomnia (Sleepiness)
Ciprofloxacin Hydrochloride Eye Drops	Ciloxan	Eye Infections
Amitriptylin	Elavil	Depression
Nortriptyline Hydrochloride	Pamelor and Aventyl	Depression

— Source: Arches of Internal Medicine via *USA Today*

Forty-Two

For the list of the five hundred "Unapproved Prescription Cough, Cold, and Allergy Products" the FDA recalled, visit

http://www.fda.gov/Drugs/GuidanceCompliance
RegulatoryInformation/EnforcementActivitiesbyFDA/
SelectedEnforcementActionsonUnapprovedDrugs/
ucm245106.htm

Below are some medications that have been said to possibly pose a potential risk to the elderly. If you or someone you know is elderly and taking the medications listed, you may want to contact the prescribing doctor and ask about possible alternatives.

Medications	Potential Side Effects
Aleve; Naprosyn (naproxen)	• abdominal bleeding • kidney damage
Benadryl (diphenhydramine)	• disorientation • overly relaxed • inability to urinate
Cardura (doxazosin)	• reduces blood pressure to low • inability to control bowel and/or bladder function

Chlor-Trimeton (chlorpheniramine)	• disorientation • overly relaxed • inability to urinate
Dalmane (flurazepam)	• disorientation • possible addiction • overly relaxed • falls
Daypro (oxaprozin)	• abdominal bleeding • kidney damage
Demerol (meperidine)	• disorientation • falls
Doral (quazepam)	• disorientation • possible addiction • overly relaxed • depression • inability to control bowel and/or bladder function
Dulcolax (bisacodyl)	• bowel problems made worst
Feldene (piroxicam)	• abdominal bleeding • kidney damage
Hytrin (terazosin)	• reduces blood pressure to low • inability to control bowel and/or bladder function
Librium or Limbitrol (chlordiazepoxide)	• disorientation • possible addiction • overly relaxed • depression • inability to control bowel and/or bladder function

Minipress (prazosin)	• reduces blood pressure to low • inability to control bowel and/or bladder function
Prozac (fluoxetine)	• agitation • sleeping problems
Sinequan (amitripty-line, doxepin)	• constipation • overly relaxed • inability to urinate
Sominex (diphenhydramine)	• disorientation • possible addiction • overly relaxed • falls
Valium (diazepam)	• disorientation • possible addiction • overly relaxed • depression • inability to control bowel and/or bladder function
Lomotil (diphenoxylate)	• possible addiction • overly relaxed

Source: "Potentially Harmful Drugs in the Elderly: Beers List and More," prescriber's letter via *Consumer Reports on Health*

Forty-Four

For those who are allergic to anesthesia, hypnosis may-be a complementary alternative. Hypnosis has been approved for medical use since 1958 and has been used in a variety of surgeries, including tumor removal. Hypnosis is considered a viable option because it has been shown to help reduce the sensation of pain and reduce recovery time. In one study, patients who received hypnosis for thyroid surgery returned to work in fifteen days compared to patients who received traditional anesthesia and returned to work in twenty-eight days.

Forty-Five

Always communicate with your doctor about any side affects you experience. If you do not communicate with your doctor, your doctor may not know what is going on. Neglecting to do so may jeopardize your overall well-being.

Forty-Six

In the words of Dr. Mike Murdock, "Establishing goals creates energy." Setting goals allow you to take something that has never existed and manifest itself into the here and now. Goals are nothing more than ideas that are powered with discipline and determination that become reality. Everything that exists today came from a goal, from cars and airplanes to televisions and cell phones. What is your idea? What goals do you have? If the answer is nothing, then it is time to reinvent yourself. Let today be the day to set your sights higher. Set a goal to start a new business, receive a job promotion, write a book, take an exotic vacation, improve your health, or anything you can think of. Whatever it is, write it down and see yourself living it daily.

When I weighed over two hundred pounds, I had a goal of having a six pack; it did not happen overnight, but I stayed with it and eventually my goal became a reality.

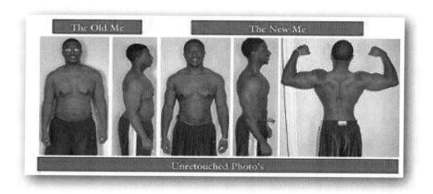

Forty-Seven

The area of the brain that is associated with memory and focusing has been shown to be 5 percent thicker in people who meditate. This is important because brain thickness may "enhance the brain's resilience against depression," according to a study published in *JAMA Psychiatry*.

Forty-Eight

The best way to destroy something is to deprive it of energy. If there is a negative experience you want to forget about, you have to stop acknowledging it. Every time an unfavorable experience is brought up, it's given new life. Everyone has made mistakes to some degree, and simply ignoring them by not thinking or talking about them and going about your day as if it never happened drains its energy. Negative experiences of any kind carry negative stress, and negative stress affects your hormones, blood pressure, body chemistry, muscles, organs, and the overall health of your body. Remember, if there is a negative or unfavorable experience you want to forget about, focus your attention on something positive and say something positive and the negative thoughts should eventually fade away.

Forty-Nine

"A happy heart is good medicine *and* a
cheerful mind works healing, but a broken
spirit dries up the bones."

(PROVERBS 17:22 AMP).

You may sometimes hear this verse of scripture translated as "Laughter doeth the body good like medicine" or "Laughter is good for the soul." Regardless of which translation you prefer, the point is the same: laughter and positive thinking promotes health and well-being. Norman Cousins put this to the test and wrote about it in his book *Anatomy of an Illness*. Norman was diagnosed with a disease in which he was given a one in five hundred chance of recovering. With the help of his doctor, Norman decided to add vitamin C, laughter, and positive thinking to his treatment regimen. What he discovered was that ten minutes of genuine laughter gave him an "anesthetic effect" and "at least two hours of pain-free sleep." Although Norman was given this slim chance of recovery, he went onto live twenty-four more years. The theory here is simple: if negativity can cause negative health reactions, then positive emotions (such as laughing and positive thinking) can produce positive health outcomes.

Fifty

If you want to have lasting change in your life, you have to change your belief system. The act of simply adopting new behaviors is known as behavior modification, and while behavior modification is beneficial, it only has temporary effects until you change your belief system. If there are aspects of your life that you know are inconsistent with living a life of honor, examine where those thoughts come from and then make it a point to renew your mind according to what is right and healthy. It may take a while, and more than likely you may face opposition, but if you renew your mind and *stick with it,* a new happier, healthier, successful you should prevail.

Renewing your mind and sticking with it, however, is the key. As Minister Creflo Dollar says, "To change your life, you have to change your mind."

"Do not be conformed to this world (this age), [fashioned after and adapted to its external, superficial customs], but be transformed (changed) by the [entire] renewal of your mind [by its new ideals and its new attitude], so that you may prove [for yourselves] what is the good and acceptable and perfect will of God, *even* the thing which is good and acceptable and perfect [in His sight for you]." Romans 12:2 (AMP).

Fifty-One

One of the easiest ways to lose weight and maintain it is to eliminate wheat from your diet. Did you know that two slices of whole wheat bread can increase blood sugar more than two tablespoons of sugar?

Wheat products (like bread, flour, cereal, pasta, noodles, bagels, and doughnuts) are counterproductive and can sabotage your weight. When you put dough or bread in the oven, it rises, and for the most part, the same is true when you put it in your body.

Fifty-Two

A sure way to maintain a healthy weight and lose excess weight is to reduce the amount of sugar you eat. When you eat or drink anything in a wrapped package or bottled container, look at its nutritional food label, typically found on the back of the packaging. There is a lot of information on nutritional labels, but do not let that discourage you. Focus your attention on the row that reads: *Sugar.* Generally speaking four grams of sugar equals one teaspoon of sugar, so if the soft drink you are drinking contains thirty grams of sugar, then you are practically consuming seven and a half teaspoons of sugar. And in case you were not aware of it, sugar is one of the leading causes of obesity.

NOTE

The sugar contents previously referred to are in reference to refined (processed) sugar; fruit and natural, 100-percent fruit juices also have sugar in them, but these are naturally occurring from the fruit itself and are not nearly as harmful.

Fifty-Three

Diet-beverage drinkers are less likely to lose weight and more likely to gain weight when compared to nondiet beverage drinkers. Diet beverages may have less sugar in them, but usually the sugar is replaced with artificial sweeteners, which tend to be much sweeter. This is a problem because the artificial sweeteners and other chemicals can trick your brain into craving more sweetness and possibly causing you to feel hungrier. And if you eat more, you are probably going to gain more. Additionally, the *Washington Post* referenced a recent study that analyzed ten years of data from people sixty five years and older and found that "the daily and occasional diet soda drinkers gained nearly three times as much belly fat as non-drinkers."

Fifty-Four

To combat the effects of sedentary behaviors like sitting and to improve overall health and function, Straighten Up America was created. The fundamental rules for performing this program are as follows:

- Think positively.
- Stand tall with confidence in the "inner winner" posture (ears, shoulders, hips, knees, and ankles all in a straight line).
- Breathe calmly, deeply, and slowly from your stomach region.
- Move smoothly; do not jerk or bounce.

NOTE
Individuals with balance disorders should use caution if attempting these exercises, and remember to always consult with your doctor before beginning any new exercise/ health regimen.

*Permission to use the Straighten Up America International Line Drawing Handout was granted by Dr. Ron Kirk of Life University.

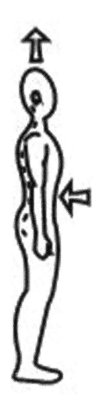

Straighten up. Stand tall in the *Inner Winner* posture. Ears, shoulders, hips, knees, & ankles should be in a straight line. Pull your belly button in towards your spine.

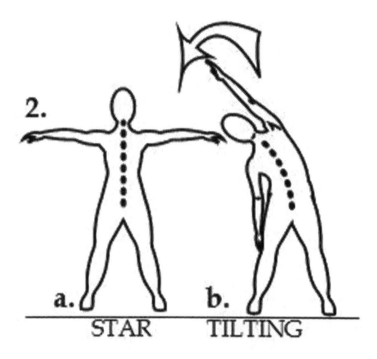

2.

a. **b.**
STAR   TILTING

From the inner winner posture, spread your arms and legs into the *Star Position* (2a).

Facing forward, place one hand in the air with the other at your side. Breathe in as you slowly stretch one arm overhead, while slowly bending your entire spine to the opposite side and sliding the other hand down your thigh (2b).

Relax at the end of the stretch, breathing out and in again. Perform slowly twice to each side.

3.

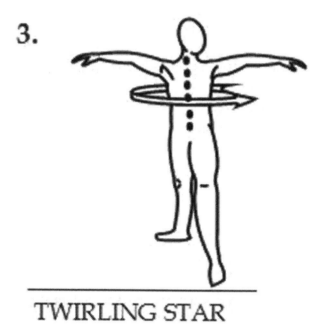

TWIRLING STAR

In the *Star Position* with your belly button drawn inward, gently turn your head to look at one hand. Slowly twist your entire spine to watch your hand as it goes behind you. Relaxing in this position breathe out and in.

Perform slowly twice to each side. Enjoy the slow, gentle stretch.

4.

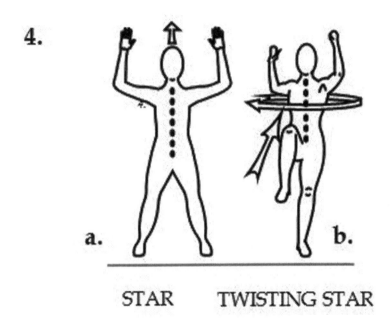

STAR   TWISTING STAR

(4a) From the *Star Position,* raise your arms in the *hands up* position.

(4b) Bring your left elbow across your torso toward your right knee. Repeat the movement using your right elbow and left knee.

Remain upright as you continue to alternate sides for 15 seconds. Breathe freely. Enjoy.

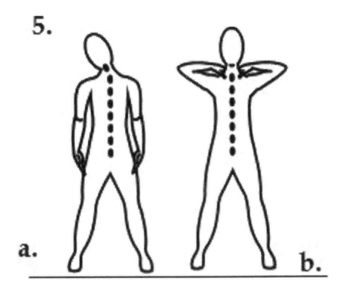

TRAP OPENERS

Breathe deeply and calmly, relaxing your stomach region.

(5a) Let your head hang loosely forward & gently roll from one side to the other.

(5b) Using your fingers, gently massage the area just below the back of your head. Move down to the base of your neck.

Then relax your shoulders and slowly roll them backward and forward. Enjoy for 15 seconds.

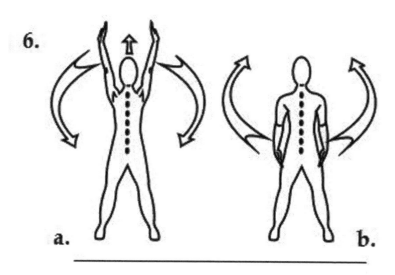

6.

a.

b.

THE EAGLE

In the *Inner Winner* posture, bring your arms out to the sides and gently draw your shoulder blades together.

(6a) Breathe in as you slowly raise your arms, touching your hands together above your head.

(6b) Slowly lower your arms to your sides as you breathe out. Perform three times.

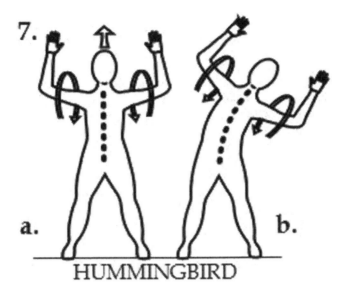

HUMMINGBIRD

(7a) Next, make small backward circles with your hands and arms drawing your shoulder blades together.

(7b) Sway gently from side to side in the *Hummingbird Position* for ten seconds.

8.

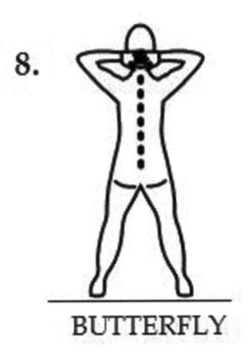

BUTTERFLY

Place your hands behind your head and gently draw your elbows backward. Slowly and gently press your head backward and resist with your hands for a count of two and release. Breathe freely. Perform three times.

Gently massage the back of your neck and head as you relax your stomach region with slow, easy breathing.

9.

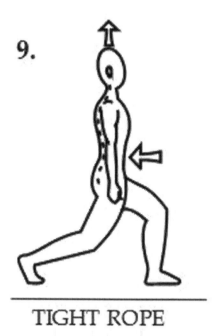

TIGHT ROPE

Stand in the *Inner Winner* position with your belly button drawn in.

Take a step forward as if on a tight rope. Make sure your knee is over your ankle & not over your toes.

Allow the heel of your back foot to lift. Balance in this position for twenty seconds. Repeat on the opposite side.

10.

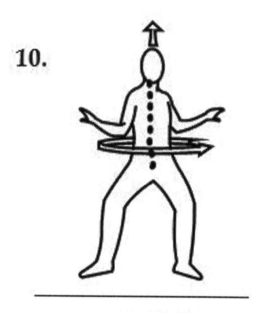

THROWING WATER

Standing tall in *Inner Winner* posture with your feet wider than shoulders, gently rotate your trunk from side to side.

Let your arms flop loosely as you shift your weight from knee to knee.

Swing gently from side to side. Breathe calmly and deeply. Enjoy for fifteen seconds.

11.

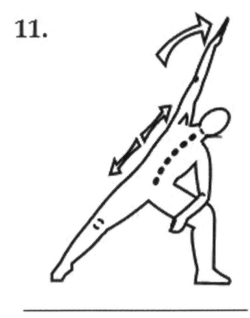

EXTENDING THE SWORD

Stand in the *Star Position*, keeping your stance wide with your belly button in.

Turn your foot outward as you shift your weight to one side. Feel the groin area gently stretching. Place your knee over ankle and elbow above your knee as you extend your arm, torso, and ribs.

(Less flexible adults should place their hand on their knee). Stretch for ten seconds to each side.

12.

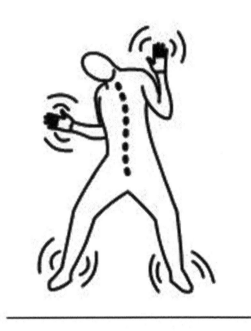

SHAKING IT LOOSE

Shake your limbs loosely for fifteen seconds.
This one is pure fun, and you are done!

**If you experience recurring or sharp pain at any time,
stop and report to your doctor. He/She may offer you
some modifications to the exercises.**

Practicing *Straighten Up America* daily has been recommended as an important feature of an active,
healthy lifestyle.

Fifty-Five

Exercising is not hard when we make it a part of our schedule rather than trying to fit it in here and there. Exercising, however, is only half the battle. The other half is staying motivated to do so. Without motivation, it is easy to get burned out and stop exercising. Staying motivated is the lynchpin to long-lasting fitness. Staying motivated to exercise and engaging in regular physical activity is something I call *Inspiration for Perspiration*.

Some inspiring strategies are as follows:

- Reward yourself.
- Schedule your workout and have a workout plan.
- Exercise in a group setting (this way your workout becomes more of a social experience than exercise).
- Listen to music as a way to distract you from the workout itself.
- Limit your workouts to less than ninety minutes: According to the American Council on Exercise, "Research shows that more than

ninety minutes of high-intensity endurance exercise can make athletes susceptible to illness for up to seventy-two hours after the exercise session."

- If you are money conscious, hire a trainer or pay for a gym membership (attaching a momentary value to your exercise routine may incentivize you to work out so that you're not wasting money).

Fifty-Six

There is no way around it: if you do not engage in some form of physical activity, the food you eat will over time result in weight gain. Did you know that just thirty-five hundred calories is equivalent to one pound of fat and that if you consume just one hundred extra calories a day for a month, you will gain close to one extra pound of fat? That may not seem like a lot, but in one year, you would have gained an extra ten pounds. When you multiply that year after year after year, the pounds will quickly add up. The recommended amount of calories that should be consumed on a daily basis varies according to age and gender, but for the most part, two thousand to twenty-two hundred calories is a good baseline (for a more accurate calculation, visit

http://www.choosemyplate.gov/weight-management-calories/calories/empty-calories-amount.html).

The key is to stay away from *empty calories,* which are calories that have close to no nutrients. As you have probably suspected, *empty calories* are typically found in breads, pastas, bagels, noodles, cereals, soft drinks, candy bars, and sugary snacks. Remember, one hundred extra calories a day can cause you to gain ten extra pounds per year.

Below is a baseline of how much physical activity is required to burn off the calories accumulated from foods that contain empty calories if you decide to eat them:

chocolate frosted donut ≈ 230 calories	59 minutes of walking
Fast-food breakfast sandwich ≈ 300 calories	32 minutes of running
large cheese pizza ≈ 320 calories	39 minutes of swimming
large fast-food french fry ≈ 540 calories	77 minutes of biking

NOTE

Simply burning off the empty calories is not enough to take your health to the next level; that just gets you back to a neutral baseline. You have to engage in more physical activity to obtain better health and optimum function. For me, having an idea of the work it takes to just burn off *empty calories* and the extra work required to become healthier makes the sugary sweets, snacks, and soft drinks not so appealing.

Fifty-Seven

As hard as we may try, our overloaded, time-consuming schedules sometimes make it nearly impossible to go to the gym. When this is the case, I suggest working out at home. One way to do this is with a kettlebell. Kettlebells can be purchased fairly inexpensively at just about any department store or sporting goods store, and best of all, you can pick it up with one hand and carry it with you just about anywhere. Free kettlebell exercises can be found on the Internet.

Another way to workout at home is by doing push-ups and sit-ups, very slowly. Many times we do things so fast that we miss the full benefits. When I am pressed for time and have to work out at home, I do push-ups and sit-ups very slowly. What I have found is that doing push-ups as slowly as I can causes me to activate the major muscles and intrinsic muscles at a higher degree, leading to a better overall workout. Doing one push-up, down and up, as slowly as I possibly can is more effective than doing five to ten push-ups quickly. Try it out, and you'll be amazed.

Fifty-Eight

Exercise and physical activity are required nutrients for the body, but the way in which those nutrients are obtained is essential. Just like with food, it is critical that your nutrients come from different sources. With advancements in fitness equipment, it seems that when it comes to strength training, *weight machines* are often times preferred over *free weights*. Exercising via weight machines can be beneficial but should not be considered the end–all, be-all or used as a regular replacement for free weights. Your body is versatile, dynamic, and designed to go through different ranges and planes of motion. Some weight machines are not. Generally speaking, weight machines move through isolated ranges and planes of motion. Only exercising in isolated ranges and the same planes of motion create muscle imbalances that can lead to injuries. Recurring isolated movements may cause your muscles to become more toned and defined, but at the expense of weakening important muscles that stabilize your joints. That is why it is advisable to use free weights in your workout routine; you develop more dynamic, functional, *real-life strength*. That way, if you happen to twist, turn, or bend awkwardly, your body will be more suitable to adapt and avoid injury.

Fifty-Nine

It has been said that a woman's life expectancy maybe increased as much as five and a half years by simply engaging in thirty minutes of physical activity five days a week.

EXERCISE MYTHS

- *No pain, no gain.* Contrary to popular belief, exercise does not and should not hurt.
- *You have to work out all day, every day.* If you are not exercising at all, thirty minutes of intense exercise three to five days a week should be sufficient.
- *Exercise has to be done in a gym.* You can bike ride, hike, dance, skate, surf, lift weights, etc. The options are almost endless.
- *Exercise is for people who want big muscles.* The human body is designed for movement. Whether you're a teenager, a centurion, or somewhere in between, there are exercises you too can do.

- *Stretch before you work out.* Stretching is a good thing, but if done at the wrong time, it can be a bad thing. We've all heard it before: "Don't forget to stretch before you work out!" Well, the truth is that you should stretch after you have warmed up. Statically, stretching (holding a stretch for twenty to thirty seconds) before warming up can possibly decrease your muscle strength by up to 30 percent.

Sixty

Yoga is an amazing way to relax and increase flexibility; however, thousands of injuries related to yoga have been reported. To reduce injuries related to yoga, consider the following:

- taking instruction from yoga instructors who are qualified and credentialed,
- informing your instructor (before class) of any illnesses and/or conditions you may have so that he or she can suggest modifications,
- wearing proper attire so that proper movement can be achieved,
- starting with the class that best suits your level and experience,
- warming up prior to class,
- asking questions if you are unsure about certain poses and positions, and
- staying hydrated.

*For more suggestions go to
http://orthoinfo.aaos.org/topic.cfm?topic=A00063

Sixty-One

Running is considered one of the most common exercises around, probably because of its ability to be done just about anywhere. However, we may be doing ourselves just as much harm as good if we run in old shoes. It is of vital importance that the shoes we wear be in good shape. As Dr. Jeffery Solomon, the president of the American Chiropractic Association's Council on Sports Injuries and Physical Fitness, explains, "Your feet are the foundation of your body, and if they are not properly supported you can have problems anywhere from the bottom of your feet up through your neck."

The entire body is connected, and the weight of all of those connected parts rest upon our feet. Each time we take a step, our feet are responsible for absorbing the impact we make when we strike the ground. And when we run, the impact can be as high as three times our body weight. As Newton explained in his third law of physics, "for every action, there is an equal and opposite reaction," so when you strike the ground, the ground transmits those forces back to you. Therefore, it is essential that your shoes be in good shape and not overworn so that your feet have a better chance of withstanding the impact and properly transferring those forces up your legs and throughout the rest of your body.

One way to determine whether your shoes are overworn is to place them on a flat surface and look and see if they are even and balanced with one another. If they are not, they are probably too old and should not be worn.

Sixty-Two

Generally speaking, shoes should have a symmetrical area across the instep where they bend upward. Shoes should not be so flexible that you can ball them up like a sheet of paper. Shoes that can be balled up may look cool, but they may be altering your biomechanics and contributing to foot pain, knee pain, hip pain, and/or low-back pain. The bend point should not be in the middle of your shoe but at the instep because that is where your foot bends.

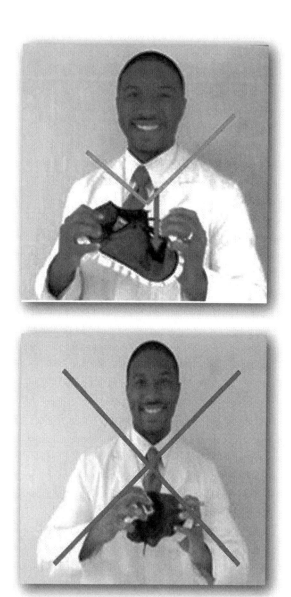

Sixty-Three

In today's society it is pretty difficult to function without the use of computer technology. That being said, there is a downfall to the technological advances we use to power our way of life. The downfall is that since we can get so much more done with the use of computers, we tend to sit in front of them way to long and develop poor posture because of it.

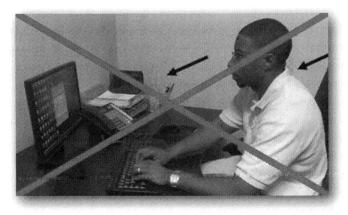

In this photo, notice how my head is leaning forward and how my upper back is hunched. This position puts undue stress on your neck and back, which can lead to headaches, neck pain, shoulder pain, back pain, sleeping problems, carpal tunnel, and double-crush syndrome.

This can be remedied by sitting more upright.

- Use a chair with a lower-back support.
- Sit with your behind pushed all the way to the back of the chair.
- Position yourself so that you are about one arm's length away from the screen, with your feet flat on the floor and your knees pointed directly at the screen. (This is also a good way to reduce excessive and improper twisting and turning.)
- Elevate your computer screen slightly above eye level so that you are looking up, not down. (You do not have to spend a lot of money to get this done; you can use phonebooks, encyclopedias, boxes, etc.)

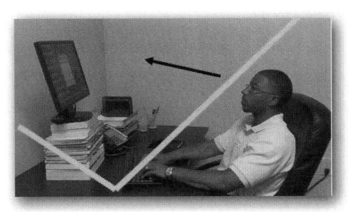

These small adjustments can help reduce headaches, neck pain, back pain, and sleeping problems.

Sixty-Four

It has been concluded that sitting for long periods of time can be detrimental to your body. In fact, the phrases commonly used in the media and health-care community(s) are "sitting is the new smoking" and "sitting disease." Did you know that it has been calculated that average Americans spend 56 percent of the time they are awake sitting? Most of the time we disregard the sitting we do as we commute to work, the sitting we do at work, the sitting we do as we commute home, and the sitting we do at home as a way of life. But in actuality sitting for eight to eleven hours a day can contribute to muscle tightness, joint stiffness, disruption in body chemistry, and increase our risk of death from all causes. Combat this by not sitting more than an hour at a time without getting up and moving around.

Add some movement into your daily sitting by:

- doing some push-ups at your desk,
- using the stairs instead of the elevator,

- sitting on a stability ball,
- squating in your chair, and
- extending your arms to your sides and rolling them forward and backward.

Sixty-Five

Back supports and braces should only be worn if your health-care professional has recommended it and/ or if you are about to lift something heavy. Back supports and braces are usually recommended for surgical recovery, fractured spines, scoliosis, and to preserve soft tissue integrity. When you wear back supports and braces when they are not necessary, you detrain your body. Just like you can train muscles to become stronger and stronger through exercise, you can also detrain muscles and their supporting structures by inhibiting them.

Each time you move, your body should engage, causing you to become stronger. However, wearing back supports and braces that are not medically necessary reduces your strength, power, energy, stamina, and overall fitness because instead of the muscles of your torso contracting to move the rest of your body, the back support and brace does the contracting for you (causing your body to become weaker and weaker). Ultimately this increases your chances of injuring yourself from everyday activities like carrying groceries and doing yard work.

As the saying goes, "if you don't use it, you lose it."

Sixty-Six

Your body functions best when things are in balance. Habits like sitting on wallets while they are in your back pocket or carrying purses in the crook of your elbow disrupts the weight distribution of your body. And when your weight is unevenly distributed, excess strain is placed on other parts of your body, resulting in aches, pains, tension, tightness, and other physiological consequences.

Sixty-Seven

Fashion trends come and go, but your health has to last a lifetime. Fashion trends like tight jeans, tight neckties, tight body shapers, and heavy purses, backpacks, and bags can cause serious health issues.

- Tight jeans can lead to nerve compression.
- Body shapers can lead to digestive problems.
- Tight neckties can lead to a reduction in blood flow to the brain.

Regarding purses, it was reported that a purse should not exceed 5 percent of a woman's body weight. That means, if you weigh 150 pounds, your purse should not weigh more than seven and a half pounds (which is about the weight of a gallon of milk). Also, be mindful of how you carry your purse, backpack, or bag. Making a simple adjustment like carrying your purse or bag on your shoulder, close to your body, as opposed to the crease of your elbow will help reduce injuries that affect your neck, shoulders, arms, wrist, and back.

Sixty-Eight

Oftentimes we dismiss car accidents with minor cosmetic damage as *fender benders*, but as it turns out, a fender bender can cause significant injuries. An accident with a speed change of as little as five miles per hour is significant enough to be deemed high risk for injury. Too often the property damage of a vehicle is used to determine how injured a person is, but this is not a great indicator. Think about a carton of eggs. Before you purchase them, you more than likely adhere to the cardinal rule of opening the carton and looking inside. You do this because you know the carton may look fine on the outside but inside the eggs could be misplaced and cracked. Well, car accidents operate in a very similar fashion. A vehicle may look fine on the outside, but the person inside the vehicle may have experienced pinched nerves, sprains, strains, and swelling from absorbing the impact of the collision. The point is that a person can be involved in a low-impact accident and still suffer injuries that can become significant if not addressed immediately. That is why I always recommend having a medical and chiropractic examination done immediately following an accident. I strongly suggest a medical exam to rule out unnoticeable life-threatening emergencies and a chiropractic exam to rule out spinal damage.

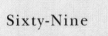

Sixty-Nine

SOME MOTOR VEHICLE
ACCIDENT EMERGENCY
SIGNS:

- battle sign: bruising or discoloration on the bony surface of the skull behind the ear lobe (possible skull fracture)

- raccoon sign: black and blue spots around the eye mimicking a black eye (possible skull fracture)

- concussion: memory loss

- pneumothorax:
  lung laceration: difficulty breathing
  rib fracture: (possible chest damage)

- joint dislocation: swelling and/or discoloration of a joint

Seventy

Everyone has the potential to save a person's life if they have the knowledge to do so. Unfortunately, this type of knowledge has not been readily available to the masses, and many people have suffered. Too often people ignore dangerous signs *and symptoms* because they think what they are going through is *normal* or due to *old age*. The Bible says that "people are destroyed for lack of knowledge," and today I want to empower you with knowledge that can be lifesaving:

Condition	Symptoms and Immediate Action
Heart Attack	• chest tightness and pain that feels like an elephant is sitting on your chest • discomfort in the jaw, neck, and arm
What to do	1. Call 911. 2. Until advanced life support arrives, the person should lay on their back with their feet elevated higher than their head.

Condition	Symptoms and Immediate Action
Stroke	• dizziness • unconsciousness • double vision or other visual problems • difficulty speaking • difficulty swallowing • walking difficulties • nausea • numbness on one side of the face and/or body • rapid eye movements
What to do	1. Call 911. 2. Until advanced life support arrives, the person's neck should be immobilized.

Condition	Symptoms
Cancer (in general)	The American Cancer Society uses the acronym **CAUTION** to identify early cancer *signs and symptoms*: • **C**hange in bowel or bladder habits • **A** sore that does not heal • **U**nusual bleeding or discharge • **T**hickening or lump in the breast, testicles, or elsewhere • **I**ndigestion or difficulty swallowing • **O**bvious change in the size, color, shape, or thickness of a wart, mole, or mouth sore • **N**agging cough or hoarseness in addition, a couple more classic cancer symptoms are as follows: • night sweats • unexplained weight loss

Seventy-One

In an issue of *Nutrition Science News*, Dr. Patrick Quillin said, "During the last 10 years, I have worked with more than 500 cancer patients as director of nutrition for Cancer Treatment Centers of America in Tulsa, Oklahoma. It puzzles me why the simple concept 'sugar feeds cancer' can be so dramatically overlooked as part of a comprehensive cancer treatment plan."

Since 1931 it has been known that cancer feeds off glucose (sugar), so a simple way to aid in cancer recovery is to eliminate sugar and sugar-forming products (like wheat) from a person's diet.

In addition to dietary modifications and treatment regimens, some cancer patients use complementary/alternative medicine (CAM) such as chiropractic care, massage therapy, and supplementation to improve their overall health.

Seventy-Two

*O*mega *6* and *omega 3* fatty acids have received a lot of press. These fatty acids are essential because among other things they are instrumental in helping the brain and body function. In your body there should be a ratio of about 1:1 or 2:1 when you compare omega 6s to omega 3s; however, because of our high consumption of vegetable oils, grains, and breads, the American ratio has been said to be as high as 25:1. This is a serious problem because high amounts of omega 6s have been linked to chronic pain, sickness, disease, and internal *silent inflammation.*

A common factor in the brains of people suffering with schizophrenia, depression, and Alzheimer's disease are low levels of omega 3 essential fatty acids. Research shows that people with higher levels of omega 3s have fewer reports of depression and negativity. Omega 3s are not made in the body and have to be obtained through food. The best source of omega 3s comes in the form of fatty fish like salmon and sardines, but because of the high levels of ocean pollution, it might be more prudent to take an omega 3 fish oil supplement. Fish oil supplements come in two forms: gel capsules and liquid oil and should:

- be distilled,
- contain natural triglyceride EPA and DHA,
- be IFOS five-star certified, and
- not taste spoiled.

I purchase mine from http://bonfirehealth.com/store/.

Seventy-Three

S upplements are wonderful but should not be taken to replace food. Instead, supplements should be taken as an added addition to a healthy diet as a way helping you become more whole and complete. Like calories, the downside to supplements and vitamins is that they are not all created equally. Like anything, there are some types of supplements and vitamins that are better than others. After the health craze hit the market, companies from all over began creating vitamins and supplements by the truckloads, some being low quality.

Biochemistry teaches us that the human body is made up of trillions of cells that undergo a variety of biochemical reactions. It is important then to make sure that the supplements we ingest are compatible with the natural biochemical reactions that occur in our bodies. When my patients ask, I suggest they take *whole food* supplements with their meals (unless otherwise indicated) rather than supplements that are *synthetically made.* The term *whole food* refers to vitamins and supplements that are primarily made from real, natural sources like plants, vegetables, and fruits and not derived from chemicals in a laboratory. *Whole food* supplements are rich in nutrients and are an easy way to give you that little extra something you may have not gotten from your daily diet. *Whole food* supplements are usually a little more expensive, but they are worth it. If you were a race car driver, you would not put economy level fuel in your car because it would not produce the performance you needed for your car to perform at its best. Furthermore, if you did put economy level fuel in your car, after a period of time, not only would your car not perform at its best, but it would also start malfunctioning and eventually breakdown. Your body is no different; it is a highly designed performance vehicle. You may have not have known this, but the human body has been calculated as being worth over $40 million, so keep that in mind the next time you purchase supplements and vitamins. Put only the best fuel in your body.

Seventy-Four

Ginseng is a plant found in Eastern Asia and North America that is used in herbal remedies. It has been suggested that it can boost the immune system and decrease the severity and lengths of multiple colds. The downside is that herbal remedies are not as regulated in America and therefore may not contain the ingredients listed on its label. Another drawback to ginseng is that it may excessively lower a person's blood pressure, but this can be combatted and/or corrected by taking ginseng with food.

Seventy-Five

As we age, bone-weakening diseases like osteoporosis become a very real topic of conversation. Lifestyle behaviors like smoking, excessive caffeine, soft drinks, and eating a diet of mostly protein should probably be avoided because of their potential of contributing to the bone-weakening process. Medications on the market can help with osteoporosis, but it has been said that a lot of people cannot deal with their side effects. A fairly inexpensive, safe alternative is strength-training exercise and walking, which can be done by just about anybody. Wolff's Law theorizes that when stress is placed on your skeletal system, your skeletal system becomes stronger as a means of stress resistance. So in other words, if you properly exercise and give yourself proper time to recover before exercising again, the stronger your bones should become.

In addition to exercising, a diet high in vegetables and fruits will help with bone strengthening. Green, leafy vegetables, broccoli, and sardines are just a few foods that are high in *absorbable calcium*. It is also important to note that just because something is labeled *high in calcium* does not mean that the calcium is readily absorbable in the body.

Seventy-Six

The increased risk of heart disease death doubles when you are deficient in vitamin D. A major cause of vitamin D deficiency is lack of outdoor activity. It is thought by many for it to be safe for fair-skinned individuals to bask in the sun without sunscreen for a few minutes, tanned individuals about fifteen minutes, and darker-skinned individuals even a few minutes longer. Having sufficient amounts of vitamin D may help fight osteoporosis, heart disease, and some cancers and may help reduce your stress.

Seventy-Seven

Belly breathing is a good way to reenergize yourself, stabilize your blood pressure, and decrease anxiety. Whenever someone is nervous, the first thing suggested is to take a deep breath. We do not make this suggestion by accident; without ever taking a college course in physiology, we just innately know that breathing deeply helps relax the body. And in the fast-paced world we live in today, it is a good idea to belly breath daily. The proper way to belly breath is to inhale in your nose while allowing your belly to push outward (as if a balloon is being inflated); then pause for a moment and slowly exhale out of your mouth while pulling your belly toward your spine. Repeating this cycle ten times in the morning is a good way to start the day.

Seventy-Eight

Sometimes we become stressed because we have so much to do and so little time to do it. It has been said that for every one minute of planning, we can potentially save ourselves six minutes of busywork. So simply taking ten minutes the night before or the morning of to plan your day might save you an hour of busywork. But the important part to planning your day is to prioritize.

List the top five things that need to be done and commit to doing them in order of complexity, with the most difficult things listed first. You want to do the most difficult things first because they usually require the most brain power and time. What most of us are used to doing is completing the easiest things on our to-do list first and then pushing the more difficult things aside and never really giving them the proper attention they need. Consequently, this adds undue stress, and our health and productivity decline as a result.

Seventy-Nine

The Message translation of Proverbs 17:22 says: "A cheerful disposition is good for your health; gloom and doom leave you bone-tired."

I heard about a pastor who, while on a hunting trip, felt somewhat down because he saw no wildlife whatsoever. So after a few hours, he packed up his things in his truck, and as he closed the trunk, he heard a loud roar behind him. When he turned around, he saw a bear standing just a few feet away. Naturally, he did the only thing he knew to do as a pastor: he prayed. He said, "Please Father, turn this bear into a Christian!" When he opened his eyes, he saw the bear raise both of his paws to the sky and say, "Thank you, Father, for the food I'm about to receive!"

The point here is to laugh. If you make it a point to laugh on a daily basis, you will have a better chance of reducing and managing stress, fight off infections, sleep better, and help your blood pressure.

Eighty

Prayer, meditation, yoga, and acupuncture are great ways to destress and rejuvenate.

Eighty-One

Once per quarter (every three months), take out time to enjoy life, revitalize, and relax. Often we burn the candle at both ends, and it is not until we are burnt out that we notice it. When this happens, you become a liability to yourself, your family, and your job instead of being an asset. To prevent burning out, plan a vacation or *staycation* every three months.

NOTE
A stay-cation is when you disconnect from the hustle and bustle of daily life and relax by engaging in activities that you do not do on a daily basis, but are within driving distance of your home.

Eighty-Two

Enduring stress on a daily basis can lead to serious health conditions like pinched nerves and ulcers. When you are frequently stressed, your body's water cycle, among other things, becomes affected. Now, instead of excreting water from your body through processes like urination, your body retains the water, resulting in an overall depletion of energy, which equals tiredness and fatigue.

Eighty-Three

Dehydration and dry, itchy skin are top subjects of conversation during the warmer months (probably due to the heighten threat of heat exhaustion). Ironically, the cooler months can lead to dehydration and skin issues as well. The fact is that when it is cold outside, we tend to sweat less and consequently become less conscious of the importance of drinking water and moisturizing our skin.

When it comes to drinking water, it is important to understand that your brain is made up of about 70 percent water and your overall body weight about 60 percent. Everyday activities like breathing, exercising, using the bathroom, drinking coffee, drinking alcohol, and taking certain medications deplete your body of water. On average men should consume about 125 ounces of total water from all beverage and food sources per day and women about 91 ounces; (with 80 percent of water being derived from liquids and 20 percent from foods). Others recommend dividing your body weight in half and consuming that amount of fluid ounces daily. (So if you weigh two hundred pounds, that calculates to one hundred ounces, or approximately twelve and a half glasses).

Eighty-Four

Fatigue, decreased concentration, and decreased alertness are all indicators of dehydration. An at-home test that can be performed to determine if you are dehydrated and not drinking enough water is to observe the color of your urine. If your urine has an odor and is not a pale yellowish color, you are probably dehydrated and not drinking enough water.

Eighty-Five

The flu is usually transmitted through inhaling, but there are times when the flu can be contracted from touching infected surfaces and then touching your eyes, mouth, or nose. A simple way to combat the flu is to wash your hands regularly and stay hydrated. Staying hydrated makes it harder for the flu virus to infect you.

Eighty-Six

If you have a problem not drinking enough water, buy a water bottle and take it with you everywhere you go. This simple strategy follows the law of propinquity. The word *propinquity* comes from the Latin word *propinquitas,* which means "nearness." In other words, the closer in proximity something is, the more inclined you are to engage it. So if not drinking enough water is the problem, simply having your water bottle in close proximity to you, where you can see it, will likely prompt you to drink more water.

Eighty-Seven

Sleeping throughout the night is a necessity, not a luxury. Staying up late not only disrupts your body chemistry and functioning ability, but it may be a big cause of weight gain. When you stay up late, not only are you typically too tired to exercise the next day, but you are also more prone to eat more because you are awake longer. A simple solution to balancing your body chemistry and maintaining a healthy weight is to sleep six to eight hours a night.

Eighty-Eight

To properly get out of bed, you should slightly bend your knees, roll to your side, and push yourself up with the free hand of the arm you are not laying on. When getting out of bed, most people bend themselves forward like they are doing a sit-up. This *sitting-up* type of motion places undue stress on your back and neck and overtime can misalign your spine and cause pinched nerves, neck pain, headaches, back pain, and strain your muscles.

Eighty-Nine

Bacteria, mildew, and fungus can harbor in pillows, so be sure to change your old pillows for new ones every two years or so.

When going to sleep, be sure not to sleep on too many pillows. When you lay down to sleep, your body should lay in a neutral position with your head centered directly over your shoulders as if you are standing straight up. Your neck is one of the most important parts of your body because all of the information coming from your brain has to first pass through your neck, and if your neck is contorted or misaligned, it may hinder your body's ability to properly function.

When you sleep, whether on your back or your side, your head should not be pushed forward, upward, or downward. This can lead to undue stress and strain, aches, pains, numbness, tingling, and even pinched nerves. This means lying on three or four pillows and reading in bed should be absolute no-nos!

Ninety

According to an article referencing the Better Sleep Council, "a good rule of thumb is to assess the condition of the mattress at least twice a year. If you're regularly waking up feeling stiff and sore after a good night's sleep, it may be time for a new mattress."

Ninety-One

An alternative to sleeping medication is a form of psychotherapy called cognitive behavioral therapy. Cognitive behavioral therapy (CBT) is where a psychologist helps retrain the portion of your brain that is associated with sleep. Participants who underwent cognitive behavioral therapy at a Veterans Affairs medical center reported having "clinically significant sleep improvements within six weeks," with some effects that lasted at least six months.

Ninety-Two

For a better night's sleep, turn off your computer, tablet, and smartphone two hours before your bedtime. These devices emit blue light, which interferes with the hormone melatonin, which is associated with sleepiness. Usually, two hours before your regular bedtime, the brain releases melatonin. The blue light from electronic devices blocks this natural process. If for whatever reason you are unable to turn off your devices two hours prior to going to bed, simply turn down the screen's brightness.

Ninety-Three

While you may be predisposed to certain health issues through your genes, your lifestyle choices, more than anything else, may determine whether those genes are turned on or not. According to the scientific journal that is published for the American Heart Association "... genetic effects are subordinate to lifestyle and environmental influences."

Ninety-Four

Lifestyle choices more than anything else determine how healthy you will be. Most illnesses are linked to how we eat, how we think, and how much physical activity we perform. It has been stated that 70 percent of illnesses are preventable.

Ninety-Five

Never, ever *pop*, *crack*, or *snap* your neck. You should consider your neck to be the most important part of your body because all of the information from your brain has to pass through it before it reaches the other parts of your body. Twisting and turning your neck because it feels tight, tense, or out of whack may start the process of arthritis and may damage your ligaments and tendons. If you take a rubber band and forcibly overstretch it, eventually it will lose it elasticity. You do not want to lose the structural integrity or elasticity in your neck due to overstretching and overstraining it. Instead, call a chiropractor who is properly qualified to adjust your neck.

Ninety-Six

The term *aromatherapy* is defined as "the use of fragrances to affect or alter a person's mood or behavior." In recent years aromatherapy has been deemed to have healing powers as well. Simply smelling certain oils and fragrances can cause a therapeutic effect within your body. The thought is that as you inhale certain aromas, your body releases chemicals that aid in normalizing your body chemistry, leading to improved health and overall well-being. Oils and fragrances are usually inexpensive and can be found at any general health food store. Some popular oils are listed below.

Oil/Fragrance	Used For
majoram	muscle cramps
eucalyptus	cough and congestion
rosemary	fatigue
lavender	insomnia (sleepiness)
ginger and peppermint	nausea

Ninety-Seven

In regards to hand sanitizer and hand washing, Allison Aiello, an associate professor of epidemiology at the University of Michigan, says, "If you can't get to a sink quickly, an alcohol-based sanitizer is a good alternative." But how long is long enough when it comes to washing your hands? Approximately twenty-four seconds, which is about the time it takes to sing "Happy Birthday" twice.

Ninety-Eight

When your body is sick and fighting something off, dairy (milk, cheese, yogurt), sugar, and wheat (breads, pastas, noodles, crackers) products may cause the infection to grow stronger. It may be counterproductive for you to eat those products when you are trying to fight some kind of infection off.

Ninety-Nine

"Gracious words are like a honeycomb,
sweetness to the soul and health to the
body."

PROVERBS 16:24 (ESV)

Researcher Dr. Masaru Emoto performed a water experiment that indicated that our thoughts, words, and feelings have power. Dr. Emoto filled bottles of water and froze them. But prior to doing so, he taped messages to the bottles, facing inward. Some of the bottles read "thank you" while others read negative words such as "you fool." What was discovered was astonishing. The bottles of water with kind words taped to them displayed the same type of "lovely" crystal formations as water that was prayed over by a priest. But the bottles of water that had negative words taped to them displayed "unpleasant, incomplete, and malformed crystals." The point is that if our thoughts, words, and feelings can affect the molecular components of water, then imagine the type of effect we place upon one another each and every day, as our bodies are made up of 70 percent water.

One Hundred

From the research of Dr. Duncan MacDougall, it is scientifically proven that our bodies possess a spiritual dimension. Prior to their death, dying patients were placed on a bed upon a weighing platform. He discovered that moments after patients died, their weight decreased, thereby scientifically proving that we possess a spiritual dimension within our physical bodies that leaves us when we die.

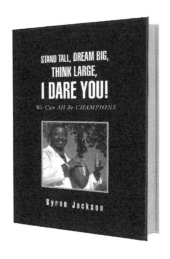

▶ **Let this powerful book help you capture the essence of what it takes to be successful!**

ISBN-10: 1425787037
ISBN-13: 978-1425787035
Price: $10.00 per copy US / Paperback
$9.50 per copy US/E-Book
Plus $3.00 shipping & handling and $1.50 shipping & handling for each additional copy.

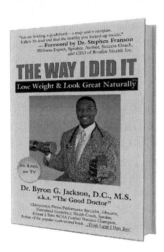

To order copies of this book, mail the form below along with payment ($10.00 per copy) plus $3.99 for shipping & handling and $2.50 for each additional copy to:
Dr. Byron G. Jackson
P.O. Box 201852
Shaker Heights, OH 44120
PH: 770-714-1157

Name: _____

Street Address: _____

City _____

State/Zip Code (required) _____

Phone: _____

TOTAL ENCLOSED $ _____

Charge Card ☐   Check/Money Order ☐

(Please make Check/Money Order payable to
Dr. Byron G. Jackson)

Card No: _____

Exp. Date: _____

Signature: _____

Note: This book is available at special quantity discounts for bulk purchase for sale promotions, premiums, fundraising, and educational needs.
Please Call 770-714-1157